THE LITTLE
BOOK OF
MARIJUANA

Mind-blowing Facts, History,
Trivia, and Recipes

An Hachette UK Company
www.hachette.co.uk

First published in Great Britain
in 2016 by Spruce, an imprint of
Octopus Publishing Group Ltd,
Carmelite House, 50 Victoria
Embankment, London EC4Y 0DZ
www.octopusbooks.co.uk
www.octopusbooksusa.com

This edition published in 2022

Copyright © Octopus Publishing
Group 2016, 2022

Distributed in the US by Hachette
Book Group, 1290 Avenue of the
Americas, 4th and 5th Floors, New
York, NY 10020

Distributed in Canada by Canadian
Manda Group, 664 Annette St,
Toronto, Ontario, Canada M6S 2C8

ISBN 978-1-84601-594-6

Printed and bound in China.

10 9 8 7 6 5 4 3 2

Standard level spoon measurements
are used in all recipes.

Eggs should be medium unless
otherwise stated.

This book includes dishes made
with nuts and nut derivatives. It
is advisable for customers with
known allergic reactions to nuts
and nut derivatives, and those who
may be potentially vulnerable to
these allergies, such as pregnant
and nursing mothers, invalids, the
elderly, babies, and children, to avoid
dishes made with nuts and nut oils.
It is also prudent to check the labels
of pre-prepared ingredients for the
possible inclusion of nut derivatives.

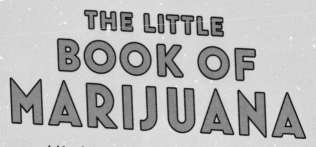

THE LITTLE
BOOK OF
MARIJUANA

Mind-blowing Facts, History, Trivia, and Recipes

CONTENTS

INTRODUCTION

Pothead, dopehead, toker, smoker, stoner, caner…
it doesn't matter what you call yourself (or what other
people call you), the fact is you love nothing more than
picking a plump pinch of bud, rolling up a nice fat
reefer and inhaling that sweet-smelling smoke.

While the herb is still shunned by lawmakers in many parts of
the world, some are gradually coming around to its qualities and
allowing their citizens to openly enjoy this most natural of highs.
Marijuana gives you a buzz that is more likely to end in a fit of
laughter than a fight; it offers relief from many medical complaints;
it offers enlightenment to religious folk; and it can be smoked or
eaten in varying quantities to achieve the desired effect.

If you've picked up this book,
chances are you're already
a fan of sweet Mary Jane
and enjoy the whole ritual of
selecting and skinning up
your weed—choosing your
variety depending on the type
of high you're looking for. Over
the following pages, we'll

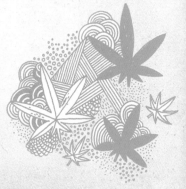

delve into the magical world of marijuana and you can extend your knowledge on building spliffs, learn about pipes and chillums, follow our step-by-step guide to making your own bong, and boost your general knowledge of marijuana movies and songs. We'll also share our survival guide to greening out and give you the lowdown on cannabis use through the ages.

So sit back, skin up a fat one, and prepare to be amazed, enlightened, and entertained as you sail away on the good ship marijuana.

WEIRD SCIENCE

THE FIVE STAGES OF A HERBAL HIGH

Everyone's different and chances are you won't feel exactly the same effects for the same length of time as everyone else in the room. And of course, your high will vary enormously depending on your choice of cheeba. But here's what you can expect to happen when you smoke a few spliffs.

1 LIFTOFF
You've been hanging out for a hit and now you've taken your first lungful of the good stuff. Bang—the world is instantly a better place.

2 BUZZING
The first few tokes will probably come in quick succession and you'll be buzzing in no time—full of energy, full of self-belief, and eventually giving in to uncontrollable laughter.

3 UTOPIA

As you settle into a long session, the initial buzz wears off and your thoughts might turn to the big philosophical questions, or how you can single-handedly achieve world peace.

4 THE INTROVERT

Keep smoking and eventually you'll run out of mind-blowing insights...or at least you'll stop sharing them with your drug buddies. Inner calm and melting-body syndrome set in, and you can literally sit or lie still for hours in a state of blissful euphoria.

5 MONGING OUT AND MUNCHIES

Even the highest high tends to peter out after a couple of hours and you'll slowly return to planet Earth with a desert mouth and an insatiable hunger.

ARE YOU STONED YET?
TEN WAYS TO TELL YOU'VE REACHED YOUR PEAK

1 YOU HAVE BECOME ONE WITH THE SOFA—YOU LITERALLY CAN'T TELL WHERE YOUR BODY ENDS AND THE CUSHIONS BEGIN.

2 YOU THINK YOU'RE STILL WATCHING THAT TELEVISION PROGRAMME THAT ENDED 20 MINUTES AGO.

3 YOU'LL EAT ANYTHING IN THE FOOD CUPBOARD THAT DOESN'T REQUIRE COOKING AND COMES IN A PACKET. HELL, YOU'LL EVEN EAT THE PACKET TOO.

4 YOUR SENSE OF HUMOR THRESHOLD BORDERS ON THE INSANE—SOMEONE SAYS "HELLO" AND YOU ROAR WITH LAUGHTER.

5 SIMPLE CONVERSATIONS LAST HOURS, AS THERE'S SUCH A HUGE GAP BETWEEN SPEAKING.

6 YOU SPEND HOURS LOOKING FOR YOUR LIGHTER...
ONLY TO FIND YOU'RE HOLDING IT.

7 THE DISCUSSIONS ABOUT WHICH TAKEAWAY TO
ORDER TURN INTO THE MOST PROFOUND DEBATES
YOU'VE EVER HAD.

8 YOU DANCE TO THE SOUND OF THE WASHING
MACHINE ON FINAL SPIN OR A CAR ALARM GOING OFF,
AND ASK YOUR MATES FOR THE NAME OF THE ARTIST.

9 YOU CAN WATCH AN ENTIRE BOX SET THEN SETTLE
DOWN THE NEXT DAY TO START IT OVER AGAIN, NOT
REMEMBERING A THING ABOUT IT.

10 COLD PIZZA, CHIPS DUSTED
WITH DOOBIE ASH, CONGEALED
CHICKEN KORMA...IT'S ALL FAIR
GAME AND MIGHTY TEMPTING
WHEN YOU'VE GOT THE
MUNCHIES.

WHAT'S GOING ON IN YOUR BRAIN?

Cannabis contains a magic ingredient called Tetrahydrocannabinol (THC), which heads straight to your brain when you smoke a spliff.

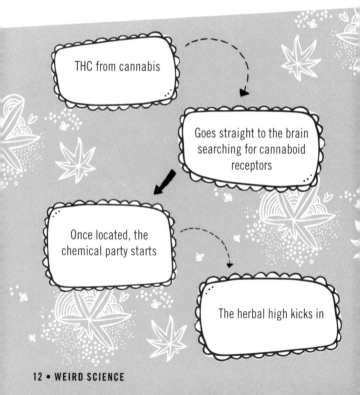

THC from cannabis

Goes straight to the brain searching for cannaboid receptors

Once located, the chemical party starts

The herbal high kicks in

20 WEIRD AND WONDERFUL MEDICINAL USES

Medicinal cannabis is legal in a number of states, but most people still have to keep their smokes out of sight. So, what exactly have cannabis campaigners throughout history claimed can be cured, dulled, numbed, and healed by the magic herb?

1 Leprosy
2 Rheumatism
3 Depression
4 Loss of appetite
5 Absent-mindedness
6 Gout
7 Muscle spasms
8 Ear pain
9 Fever
10 Dysentery
11 Constipation
12 Convulsions
13 Insanity
14 Sexual desire
15 Nausea
16 Colic
17 Kidney stones
18 Impotence
19 Tetanus
20 Bronchitis

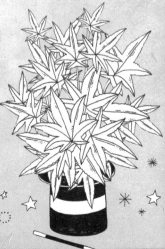

THE HERB IN HISTORY

CANNABIS TIMELINE:
TOP TOKING CULTURES THROUGH THE AGES

When you're flying on a cannabis high, it's easy to think you're the first person to discover this wonder plant and that no one else in history could possibly have felt as good as you do now. But don't be fooled—people have been enjoying the fruits of this forbidden plant for many thousands of years.

The first recorded use of cannabis goes way back to 6000 BC but that's just as far back as some archeologist dude could trace some seeds—there were probably generations of stoners before that who were too busy enjoying a smoke to think about leaving a record for the history books.

2700 BC

Someone discovers that cannabis is a wonder drug and it's widely adopted as a medicinal plant.

6000 BC

China leads the way by including cannabis seeds in meals.

4000 BC

We're back in China, and this time people are making clothes from hemp.

1200 BC

The Egyptians jump on the bhang bandwagon and prescribe cannabis for a whole host of medical horrors.

1000 BC

Medicinal marijuana hits the big time in India.

200 BC

We're off to Ancient Greece now where the doctor's notepads are crammed full of cannabis prescriptions.

AD 79

Pliny the Elder, the Roman writer, gives cannabis the scientific thumbs-up when he pens about the positive virtues of pot in his life's work *Naturalis Historia*.

AD 30

Even Jesus wasn't immune to the potency of pot, as he apparently douses his followers in cannabis oil.

1611

Early American settlers pack up some pot plants in their luggage and set about cultivating it for export.

1850

Marijuana gets official recognition in the US when it's added to pharmacy shelves as a treatment for everything from insanity to alcoholism.

1913

California spoils the pot party when it passes an anti-marijuana law, with other states joining in soon after.

HIGH ACHIEVERS:
FAMOUS SMOKERS FROM HISTORY

SHAKESPEARE

They say that cannabis use can heighten creativity, so if the rumors are true and Shakespeare was a toker, that's a pretty good argument for lighting up. Apparently, someone dug up some 17th-century pipes in the bard's backyard that contained traces of cannabis.

ABRAHAM LINCOLN

It seems that many a president liked to get high while in high office—the 16th President of the United States was alleged to have enjoyed the odd smoke on his veranda.

QUEEN VICTORIA

Ruler of the British Empire from 1837 until 1901, Queen Vic couldn't let painful monthly menstrual cramps stand in the way of the expansion of the British Empire. So her private physician, Sir Russell Reynolds, prescribed marijuana in 1823 to ensure PMS wouldn't cramp her style.

CHRISTOPHER COLUMBUS

In 1492 this Italian explorer first sailed to the New World under the patronage of the Spanish crown, and was responsible for carrying *Cannabis sativa* seeds to America. Some people suspect he may have enjoyed a few cheeky spliffs en route to assuage his concerns about sailing off the edge of the world.

GEORGE WASHINGTON

Did he strike up a blunt while pondering great political conundrums? Well, the jury's still out on whether he was an avid smoker, but he certainly grew plenty of hemp and sold it for industrial use.

OSCAR WILDE

The doomed writer wrote about cannabis and was believed to dabble in the odd spliff, although he generally preferred to release his creativity by drinking absinthe.

BOB MARLEY

The king of skinning up—you'll be hard-pressed to find a photograph of the famous reggae artist without a spliff in his hand.

FOR THE GREATER GOOD:
FIVE RELIGIONS THAT USE THE HERB

1 RASTAFARIANISM

The holy herb is held in high reverence by Rastafarians and is smoked for spiritual enlightenment (who doesn't get a bit deep and meaningful after an evening on the good stuff?). Gatherings involve music and meditation, so not unlike a Saturday night with your mates and a bag of doobie. And best of all there's often a shed-load of food, which is just as well, as a roomful of spiritual stoners are going to have the mother of all munchies.

* HERBAL RATING 9/10

2 HINDUISM

Anyone who's taken the well-worn traveler path to India will appreciate the reverence of the herb in Hinduism. The holy men, or sadhus, get their spiritual nourishment by toking on clay pipes called chillums. Not for the fainthearted, these are essentially huge tubes packed full of high-grade weed. If you're not sitting down when you go in for a toke, you'll be knocked off your feet and flat on your behind once you've puffed. It is believed that the god Shiva was so grateful for the shade provided by a mighty cannabis plant on a sweltering day that he donated it to the human race as a thank you gift...other religions take note!

* HERBAL RATING 7/10

3 THE ETHIOPIAN ZION COPTIC CHURCH

Touted by some as a cover-up for a bunch of people getting high in the name of God, this is actually a fully-fledged and recognized religion that just happens to hold the herb very dear to its spiritual heart. Followers of the religion believe God put marijuana on Earth for everyone to enjoy—and they certainly do enjoy it, sparking up throughout the day in between chanting. This religion is seriously devoted to its weed.

HERBAL RATING 8/10

4 TAOISM

The ancient Chinese were no strangers to the wonders of marijuana. Its hallucinogenic properties were highly prized as a way to chat to the spirits, rather like an old-school social media chat room. Hemp is mentioned in Taoist texts dating back to the 6th century, so weed use in the religion wasn't just word of mouth. As Taoism centered on taking a stress-free path through life and choosing the easy option, it seems pretty fitting the cannabis plant would have a part to play.

HERBAL RATING 6/10

5 SIKHISM

Bhang (a marijuana preparation) has been part of the Sikh religion for much of its history, with warriors indulging after battles, presumably to have a bit of a chill-out session after a hard day evading death. But there's always been a bit of banter among the top bods in the religion as to whether the mighty herb aids spiritual awareness or makes people lose focus of the Divine.

HERBAL RATING 5/10

KNOW YOUR BLOW

WHAT'S YOUR STRAIN?

Any decent dopehead will have a couple of bags of their favorite weed on hand for a mid-morning pick-me-up or mellow, midnight smoke. The beauty of the herb is that you can pick a strain to suit your mood—from getting wired to chilling out. For the purposes of conserving brain cells, let's stick to the basics.

SATIVA

These plants can grow as high (see what we did there?) as a house and the delicate leaves are the universal symbol for pot. If you've spent a night on the indica, then a hit on a sativa spliff is what you need the next morning to give you a burst of energy and to kick-start your day enough to get your butt out of bed.

INDICA

If you want to hit the wall and lose control of your mind and limbs, then pick an indica. These short plants are popular with home-growers, but save your indica smoking for late-night sessions, as you won't be going anywhere fast after a couple of blasts on these spliffs.

HYBRIDS

Over the years, pot lovers have created blends that take the best bits of indica and sativa strains to create new varieties of weed—so you can quite literally have your cake and eat it. They've tweaked and toked on your behalf so you can choose a very specific smoke with a flavor, aroma, and buzz to float your boat. Of course, you can also create your own blends by mixing together a couple of different varieties to fill your spliff.

20 GREAT SMOKES
TO BLOW YOUR MIND

Here's our pick of the pot—varieties to fire you up
or knock you flat on your back.

NAME	STRAIN	BUZZ	FLAVOR
Maui Waui	SATIVA	Mild/medium	SWEET
Panama Red	SATIVA	Intense, happy	STRONG, EARTHY
Purple Haze	SATIVA	Intense	EARTHY
Jack Herer	SATIVA	Intense	EARTHY, WOODY
Shipwreck	SATIVA	Medium	SPICY
Kali Mist	SATIVA	Medium	SWEET, NUTTY
Sour Diesel	SATIVA	Medium/intense	DIESEL

NAME	STRAIN	BUZZ	FLAVOR
Blueberry	INDICA	Medium	SWEET BERRY
Hollands Hope	INDICA	Medium/intense	FRUITY
Purple Kush	INDICA	Intense	SWEET
Grandaddy Purple	INDICA	Intense	SWEET BERRY
Blackberry Kush	INDICA	Medium	SWEET BERRY
G13	INDICA	Intense	SWEET
Northern Lights	INDICA	intense	SWEET
Bubba Kush	INDICA	Intense	EARTHY
Girl Scout Cookies	HYBRID	Intense	SWEET
Cherry Pie	HYBRID	Long high	CHERRY
White Widow	HYBRID	Happy	EARTHY
Mango Kush	HYBRID	Uplifting	MANGO
Orange Diesel	HYBRID	Euphoric	SWEET CITRUS

WHAT'S YOUR FAVORITE FLAVOR?

If you're more concerned with the flavor of your spliff than the effects of the high, you can pick your bag of bud based on flavor and aroma. Do you fancy wafts of vanilla smoke swirling around your bedroom? No problem, score yourself some Willy Wonka.

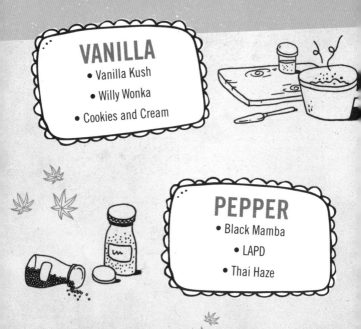

VANILLA
- Vanilla Kush
- Willy Wonka
- Cookies and Cream

PEPPER
- Black Mamba
- LAPD
- Thai Haze

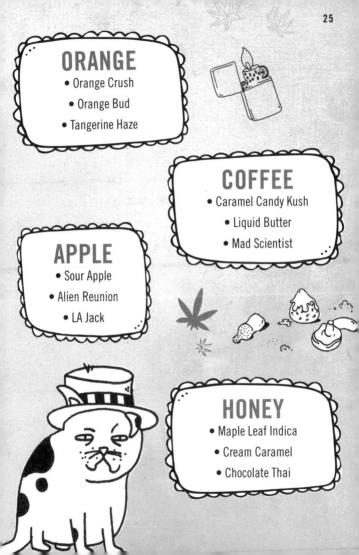

ORANGE
- Orange Crush
- Orange Bud
- Tangerine Haze

COFFEE
- Caramel Candy Kush
- Liquid Butter
- Mad Scientist

APPLE
- Sour Apple
- Alien Reunion
- LA Jack

HONEY
- Maple Leaf Indica
- Cream Caramel
- Chocolate Thai

EMERGENCY EXIT:
FIVE REMEDIES FOR GREENING OUT

We've all been there—taking a few too many hits on a spliff that was loaded with some heavyweight bud. The important thing is not to panic. Sure, you or your green buddy will feel like poo on a stick for the next few hours…and possibly the next day…but there are a few surefire ways to bring your brain and body back down to Earth and make you feel vaguely human again.

1

FIND A QUIET SPACE
Loud conversations, music, and bright lights can add to the confusion, so walk, crawl, or drag yourself somewhere quiet to begin your recovery.

2

REHYDRATE
Smoking gives you a thirst and if you've been on the hard stuff, who knows when you last had a sip of something non-alcoholic. Ask a mate to get you some water and sip it slowly (too fast and it might come straight back up).

3 BREATHE

Serious greenouts can result in panic attacks and irregular breathing, so try to take slow, controlled breaths in and out while you get your head together.

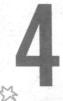

4 FRESH AIR

When you panic you tend to overheat, so getting some fresh air can help to cool you off and calm you down.

5 SLEEP IT OFF

If you can make it to bed, then this is the best place to recover. It's familiar, safe, and comforting and you won't freak out if you wake in the night in a strange place.

TOKER'S TOOLBOX

Every self-respecting stoner needs a drawer full of gadgets to make life that little bit easier when it's time to roll up a fat one. You'll no doubt have your own techniques and routines when it comes to skinning up, but here's the lowdown on some of the essential kit to help you get high.

ROLLING PAPERS

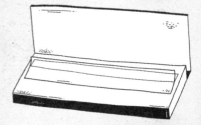

The novice stoner will be overwhelmed by the sheer variety of rolling papers on the market—long, short, extra large, extra thin, organic, flavored. But as you ease yourself into the art of rolling you'll get a feel for the type of paper you prefer and the brand that does the best job. Try out a few different varieties and see how they smoke—everything is available online, so there's no excuse to get caught short.

STASH TIN

Everyone has one
—it might be a
dented old box
with sentimental
value or a swish
new tin that's been
purchased with the
sole purpose of stashing
your gear. Whatever it is, keep
it stocked with a good supply.

ROLLING MAT

These take the fear factor out of the art of rolling by giving you a
helping hand at the crucial stage of creating your spliff. They're
cheap and are often made of bamboo, which means they're also
lightweight and easy to store and transport. No matter how steady
your hand, this is an essential addition to your kit if you want to
steer clear of baggy spliffs that won't last a round of tokes.

ROACHES

Gone are the days when your used train ticket had to double
up as roach paper. With packs of roaches that have been specially
designed for the job, you can put the finishing touches to your spliff
with a little finesse. As with rolling papers, there are different sizes
and thicknesses available, and roach research is the ideal excuse
for an extended smoking session.

OTHER WAYS TO SMOKE

When it comes to getting high, you don't always have to reach for the rolling papers and roaches. Sometimes a regular roll-up just isn't going to cut it—you might have a few friends round for a stoner's sit-in or your fingers aren't feeling dexterous enough to create a cone. There are plenty of options available for anyone who's too stoned or lazy to skin up. This is when bongs, chillums, and pipes come into their own.

PIPES

If you like the idea of sitting in front of a log fire in your slippers, with a dog and a glass of whiskey by your side, a pipe might be the smoking vessel for you. As with bongs, pipes are available in very simple or ornate styles and in a variety of materials. The good thing about these little beauties is that they can slide into a back pocket without anyone suspecting they're walking behind a caner. And there's no need to keep a constant supply of rolling papers and roaches in the house—just fill your pipe and smoke it.

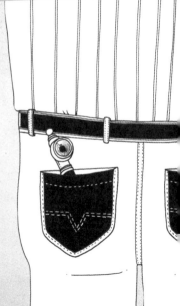

CHILLUMS

The favored way for holy men to get their daily hit, these conical pipes are usually made from stone or clay. If they're good enough for reefer-loving Rastafarians, they're good enough for any self-respecting stoner.

BONGS

Bongs work by filtering the smoke through water in the bowl. This results in a very smooth smoke and can be less harsh on your throat.

Bongs are available in such a vast array of styles and materials that it's sometimes too much for the average stoner to decide which one to buy. A lot of it will come down to budget and how much you're willing to spend, but you should be able to pick up a fairly decent basic bong for under $20. And if you're really strapped for cash, you can always make your own (see pages 32–35).

Bongs can be anything from small, simple, single-tube systems to massive, multi-chamber behemoths that most removal guys would charge double time to shift. Once you've decided whether you want to be able to tuck your bong in your daypack or would rather install it as a piece of permanent furniture in your den, it's time to decide on which material, and there's plenty to choose from:

- ACRYLIC Standard-issue acrylic bongs are cheap and fairly hardwearing.
- GLASS Make sure it's reinforced glass for obvious reasons!
- CERAMIC If you choose carefully, your short-sighted elderly aunt might mistake this for an ornament.
- WOODEN These are usually made from bamboo and can be very simple or feature elaborate designs.
- METAL A good choice for clumsy caners as these are virtually unbreakable.

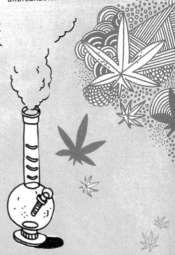

BUILD YOUR OWN BONG

So, you're at a loose end on a Saturday morning (or more likely afternoon if you've been getting hold of some serious-grade weed for Friday night smoke-ins). There's nothing on TV, your mates are still snoring in their pits, and the liquor store doesn't open for another hour. Why not make the most of this unexpected free time and make a bong?

A bong is essentially a bowl and a pipe, and the great thing is it can be made out of virtually anything (note the "virtually" here). So, that means you probably don't need to change out of your trackie pants and leave the house; you can search through the garbage and probably find all you need. Plastic water bottles, chip cartons, cans, bits of pipe—if you can cut a hole in it and it's not likely to melt or disintegrate, then chances are you can make it smoke.

Here's our step-by-step guide to building a badass bong that will make your house the go-to venue for smoking sessions. You can get as creative as you like, but we're keeping things fairly simple here for your first attempt, and assuming standard trashcan contents.

WHAT YOU NEED

- Scissors

- Empty plastic bottle (don't worry if the lid is missing, as you won't need this)

- Pipe (this can be a piece of plastic or metal tube, or a pen shaft)

- Duct tape

- Bowl (from a smoking shop), or rolling papers

BUILD YOUR OWN BONG
CONTINUED...

HOW YOU MAKE IT

1   Very carefully cut a hole about 2 inches from the bottom of the bottle. The hole should be just big enough to fit the pipe.

2   Push the pipe through the hole so that it's angled down into the base of the bottle but not touching the bottom.

3   Seal around the pipe with duct tape. This needs to be as airtight as possible so you get the benefit of all the smoke.

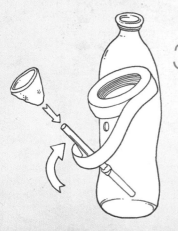

4 Fix the bowl to the end of the pipe to hold the weed. If you don't have a bowl at home you can make one from rolling papers and put the end inside the top of the pipe.

5 Pour water into the bottle until the bottom of the pipe is covered by about 1 inch of water.

6 Next, make a small air hole about halfway down the bottle, on the other side from the pipe but above the water line. This lets oxygen into the bong.

7 Fill the bowl with weed, spark it up and suck in the smoke from the top of the bong, covering the air hole while you smoke.

A–Z OF AMSTERDAM COFFEE SHOPS

A trip to the Netherlands should be on every stoner's travel itinerary, but unless you decamp to the country permanently you're unlikely to be able to visit every coffee shop on the block. With so many to choose from, it's best to just pick the name you like the sound of, or a shop front that looks welcoming and head on inside…you might be some time.

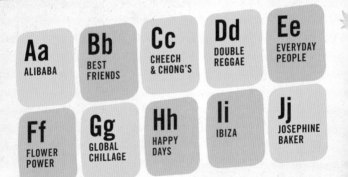

Aa ALIBABA

Bb BEST FRIENDS

Cc CHEECH & CHONG'S

Dd DOUBLE REGGAE

Ee EVERYDAY PEOPLE

Ff FLOWER POWER

Gg GLOBAL CHILLAGE

Hh HAPPY DAYS

Ii IBIZA

Jj JOSEPHINE BAKER

Kk KIF KIF

Ll LUCIFERA

Mm MARIMBA

Nn NATTY CULTURE

Oo OLD AMSTERDAM

Pp PINK FLOYD

Qq*

Rr RISKY BUSINESS

Ss SPACE MOUNTAIN

Tt TOMORROW-LAND

Uu UTOPIA

Vv VOYAGERS

Ww WHEN NATURE CALLS

Xx*

Yy YELLA

Zz ZONNETJE

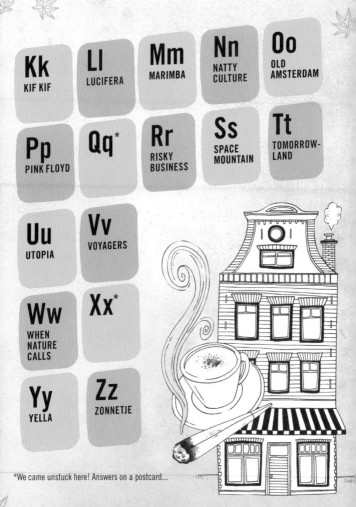

*We came unstuck here! Answers on a postcard...

TOP TIPS FOR COFFEE SHOP NEWBIES

If you do make a pilgrimage to the spiritual home of cannabis, there's a few things to consider before you swing the doors open, make your way through the fog of smoke, and order an ounce of finest marijuana.

KNOW YOUR JARGON

A coffee shop is a cannabis retailer but a *koffiehuis* is definitely not (this is where you go if you actually want a cup of caffeine). Licensed coffee shops have a distinctive white and green poster in the door or window to avoid confusion and embarrassment.

READ THE MENU

You'll find different menus in every coffee shop and there's going to be varieties you've never heard of. Ask for advice and take it slowly—it's easy to act like a kid in a candy store and order one of everything...do that and you won't come around until it's time to fly home. Amsterdam weed is pretty potent anyway, so start off with something light and work your way towards the stronger varieties.

PRICE PER GRAM

Most coffee shops in Amsterdam sell cannabis by the gram and a general rule of thumb is that the pricier it gets, the stronger it is. You can legally buy up to 5 g (about ⅕ oz) per day, which should be more than enough, even for the most seasoned smoker.

YOU WANNA BEER WITH THAT?

It recently became illegal for coffee shops in Amsterdam to sell alcohol as well as cannabis, so bad luck if you like to suck on a cold Bud while you smoke your spliff. You'll have to go to a bar for your beer hit afterwards, if your legs still work after a few hours in a coffee shop.

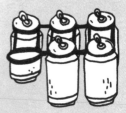

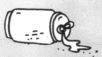

SKINNING-UP SKILLS

DIY ROACH

The roach keeps the joint stable and stops it getting soggy and sealing up. Sure you can buy ready-made roaches in neat little packs along with your papers, but why bother when you can make your own for free? Here's how.

1 Choose thin card, ideally plain and not glossy.

2 Cut a piece about 2 x 1 inches (cut out at few at the same time so you've got a ready supply).

3 Gently roll the card between your thumb and forefinger so it forms a coil. You want it to have enough substance to stop the weed escaping but not so many rolls that you can't smoke the spliff—practice makes perfect.

Some people prefer to roll the roach up nice and tightly, slot it into the business end of the spliff, and let it gently unwind until it fits like a glove. Others prefer to roll the spliff around the roach to create a more tailored finish. There's no right or wrong way, you'll find your own rolling groove.

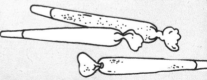

FIVE STEPS TO BUILDING
A CONE, A BLUNT, AND A TULIP

Technically, a spliff is a pure-weed smoke, whereas a joint is a combination of cannabis and tobacco. But whether you like yours pure or mixed up a little, the rolling techniques are the same.

THE CONE

This is the classic spliff that you need to master if you intend to smoke among friends. Practice on your own until you're confident enough to roll in front of an audience, and always use good-quality papers.

1 Lick and stick two rolling papers together at a 45° angle.

2 Add the roach to the horizontal paper and pack in the weed along the middle of this paper.

3 Begin carefully rolling from the horizontal paper, working at an angle to create a cone shape as you roll, and sticking the first paper down.

4 Now work the rest of the remaining paper, packing down the weed and creating a nice tight spliff.

5 Neaten up the edges, twist the top, and spark up.

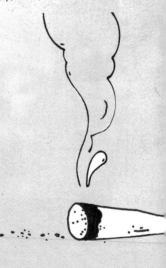

5 STEPS TO BUILDING
A CONE, A BLUNT, AND A TULIP CONTINUED...

THE BLUNT

This is basically a hollowed-out cigar that's filled with the good stuff. It means tokers can take their smokes outside without looking (too) dodgy and the cigar paper also adds an extra flavor dimension to the smoke.

1 Using a sharp knife, carefully cut along the length of the cigar to split it open.

2 Remove the tobacco and replace it with your weed or combo mix.

3 Starting at one end, roll the blunt really tightly to pack in the weed and create an overlap of the cigar paper.

4 Lick the underside of the paper as you go—this can be fiddly, but take your time and roll each section firmly so the paper sticks.

5 Keep working your way along the blunt until you have rolled, licked, and glued the entire paper. Enjoy!

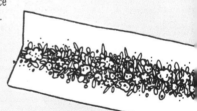

THE TULIP

Once you've mastered the basic cone, it's time to move onto more creative spliffs, and the tulip is a real showstopper. It brings together two of the things Holland is most famous for: weed and tulips. This one will knock your socks off, as the hit gets progressively stronger as the bulb gets wider.

1 Overlap two big papers to form a square and create a regular straight joint with a small roach at one end, then add a second larger roach at the other end.

2 Make another square with two papers and fold the upper, right-hand corner of the square over towards the lower, left-hand corner. Lick the gummed edge and seal it to create a cone shape.

3 Fill the cone two-thirds full with a mix of weed and tobacco, and push it down gently towards the tip of the cone.

4 Pull together the excess paper at the top of the cone and put the end of the spliff with the larger roach inside.

5 Scrunch the paper tightly around the roach and tie a piece of string or an elastic band around it so that the cone is tightly sealed to the spliff.

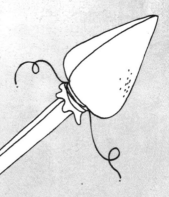

WINDMILL

So-named because yes, you've guessed it, it looks like a windmill. You're basically getting four joints in one hit with this bad boy so take it slowly, as a couple of tokes will give you a huge high. This one isn't for beginners and you need to master the art of basic rolling before you even consider giving this a try.

JOKER

This is essentially the biggest badass spliff you'll ever roll, so make sure you've got a few mates handy to help you smoke your way through it—this is so much more than a one-person job. The joker is a five-paper spliff, which tells you all you need to know about its size and the length of time you'll be sitting on the sofa after smoking it.

CROSSROADS

This spliff is basically a three-way roach
that is built to be re-used. The beauty of this
creation is that you can pick three different joints
to smoke at the same time so you can be creative with
flavor and strength combinations, and find the ideal mix.

SECRET AGENT

Also known as a "spliferatte" this is one for potheads
who need a hit on the go without attracting unwanted
attention. Easy enough to create, you simply replace
a cigarette filter with a roach and then snip away
half the cigarette, empty the tobacco, and fashion
your spliff around the stump. Alternatively, you can
carefully empty out the cigarette and fill it with weed.

MIND-BENDING FACTS

THE A–Z OF CRAZY WEED NAMES

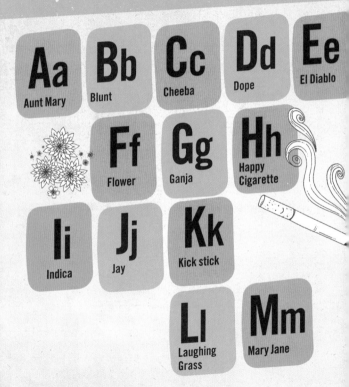

Aa Aunt Mary

Bb Blunt

Cc Cheeba

Dd Dope

Ee El Diablo

Ff Flower

Gg Ganja

Hh Happy Cigarette

Ii Indica

Jj Jay

Kk Kick stick

Ll Laughing Grass

Mm Mary Jane

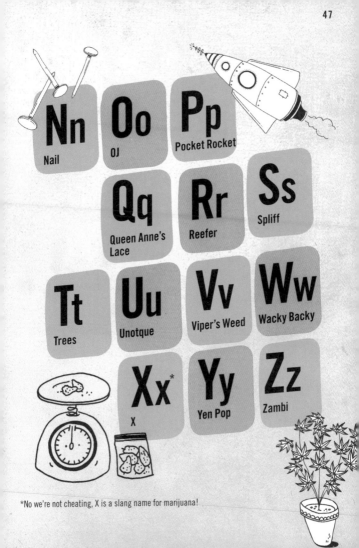

Nn Nail

Oo OJ

Pp Pocket Rocket

Qq Queen Anne's Lace

Rr Reefer

Ss Spliff

Tt Trees

Uu Unotque

Vv Viper's Weed

Ww Wacky Backy

Xx* X

Yy Yen Pop

Zz Zambi

*No we're not cheating, X is a slang name for marijuana!

POTHEAD TRIVIA

- Over 22 million people worldwide smoke pot every day.

- Marijuana is the most used illegal drug in the US.

  - Eating cannabis gets you higher than when you smoke it.

    - You can't get high on hemp.

  - Cannabis is America's biggest cash crop.

- 20% of US high-school kids admit to regularly sparking up a spliff.

- The average cannabis plant grows 1–2 inches a day.

- In 1913, California became the first state to ban marijuana.

- In a weird cyclical twist, in 1996 California then became the first state to legalize medical marijuana.

- In Italy, Rastafarians can legally possess marijuana on religious grounds.

- Beer is a distant relation to marijuana— hops are in the same plant family.

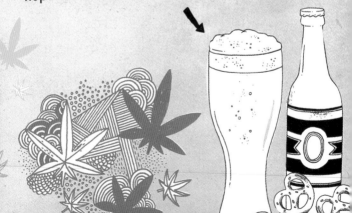

STUPIDEST SMUGGLING ATTEMPTS

Sometimes you feel like you'd do anything for a toke on a doobie, but count your lucky stars that you never did something as stupid as these desperados.

• Colombian drug smugglers tried to pull a fast one on the border patrol by going off radar. They used a homemade submarine to float their stash to its destination.

• Catapults are regularly used to fire packages of cannabis from Mexico into the US...with varying degrees of success.

• Sticking with the Mexican border, other ingenious (or should we say stupid) ideas for getting marijuana consignments Stateside have included canons, torpedoes, and lightweight homemade aircraft...some people have way too much time on their hands.

• How about a weed-filled wheelchair? That's how one man tried to get his stash through customs. Needless to say he was caught.

• Christmas is a major celebration in Germany, and one herbal enthusiast was hoping for an especially good time when he decorated an enormous cannabis plant with lights and baubles. The police didn't share his festive spirit and put a dampener on the celebrations when they arrested him.

• One drug smuggler put his creative talents to the test when he painstakingly painted large balls of tightly wrapped marijuana to look like watermelons traveling to market in the back of a truck. Unfortunately, he must have skipped a few of his college lectures, as his efforts weren't good enough to get past US customs.

• Over the years, a number of women have upped a few cup sizes on international trips, as they've stuffed their bras full of bags of weed.

• It's said that humans have a special bond with animals, and this is particularly true of carrier pigeons. A Colombian pigeon trainer put this bond to the test when he strapped a consignment of weed to his bird and sent it on a delivery mission to his mates in the local jail. They were waiting patiently by the window for the arrival of the bird, but unfortunately for them, so were the prison wardens.

20 THINGS YOU NEVER KNEW WERE MADE FROM HEMP

Hemp is a variety of cannabis that won't get you stoned, but as a close relative of the herb in your spliff, it's a pretty important player in the marijuana PR race.

As one of the most versatile natural resources on our planet, it's no great surprise that humans discovered this miracle plant many thousands of years ago and soon began turning it into all manner of materials to make ancient life more tolerable.

1 **PAPER**
2 **CLOTHES**
3 **PLASTIC**
4 **MILK SUBSTITUTE**
5 **ROPE**
6 **INK**

7   **FIBERBOARD**

8   **ANIMAL FEED**

9   **FLOUR**

10   **SHAMPOO**

11   **CEMENT BLOCKS**

12   **ICE CREAM**

13   **FUEL**

14   **LIP BALM**

15   **CARPET**

16   **CANVAS**

17   **COOKING OIL**

18   **VARNISH**

19   **DISH CLOTHS**

20   **WAX**

LIGHT UP LEGALLY

Different countries have very different attitudes to possessing and smoking the holy herb: here's our lowdown on some potential holiday destinations for potheads.

NETHERLANDS

The country's coffee shops do a roaring trade in cannabis, but these are the only places where it's legal to buy the drug.

JAMAICA

With its Rasta culture and Bob Marley as its favorite son, it would seem criminal to criminalize cannabis here. But while possession of very small amounts has been decriminalized, it's still illegal to sell and use cannabis.

ECUADOR

If you're caught with under 10 g (about ⅖ oz) and you can prove it's for personal use, you'll be let off the hook in this forward-thinking South American country.

COLOMBIA

Things are even better here—you can grow up to 20 plants for personal use and possess up to 22 g (about 1 oz) of cannabis without breaking the law.

PORTUGAL

In 2001, Portugal was the first country to legalize drugs. But if you're a repeat user you might be sent to rehab, so it's always better to toke behind closed doors.

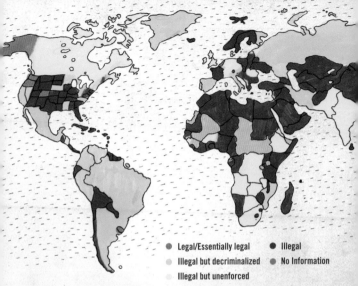

Legend:
- ● Legal/Essentially legal
- ● Illegal but decriminalized
- ● Illegal but unenforced
- ● Illegal
- ● No Information

SPAIN

Head across the Portuguese border and you're also fairly well looked after as a pothead. There's a bit of a grow-your-own culture emerging here, with authorities turning a blind eye to people growing and using their own pot in private. However, step outside with your spliff and the law will be waiting.

US

We're catching up with some of the more lenient locales, with Washington, Oregon, Alaska, and Colorado states legalizing recreational use, while others have relented to medicinal use.

WORLD'S CRAZIEST DRUG BUSTS

If you're meticulous about hiding your stash out of sight of prying eyes, take a moment to consider these ambitious and downright crazy smuggling attempts—there's no way these hauls were ever going to fit under the mattress.

In 2010, Mexican authorities set fire to a massive pile of marijuana with a street value of $435 million. It took two days to burn the stash—there must have been some seriously caned passersby.

In 2008, the UK's Royal Air Force Harrier jets dropped three massive bombs on a 237-ton haul of cannabis in a desert in Afghanistan. The weed was worth over $350 million.

A seizure of 20 tons of marijuana off the coast of Italy in 2013 was believed to be the biggest drug bust ever made at sea.

Drug smugglers must have thought their canny idea to fill 1,000 olive cans with cannabis was a winner...until Irish police intercepted the haul on its way to the UK. Now that would have made for an interesting pizza topping.

In January 2015, Arizona police intercepted a truck stuffed with $3 million worth of marijuana. It turned out the truck had picked up its haul from the entrance to a cross-border tunnel that stretched over 905 ft, the longest discovered on this notorious stretch of underground weed routes between Mexico and the US.

Arizona was also the location for possibly the weirdest way to try to get drugs past border patrol. Smugglers attached a trailer to an off-road buggy and made it to within yards of the border before doing a runner when they were spotted.

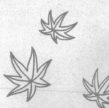

THE BIG NIGHT IN

GANJA GAMES

A night on the smokes isn't always the most sociable way to hang out with your buddies. As soon as a couple of generously proportioned spliffs have done the rounds, the art of conservation is either lost to deadly silence or inane giggling. So, if you want to inject some action into your evening, try out one of our ganja games, guaranteed to drag even the most comatose caner back to reality…at least for a few minutes.

BLINDFOLDED JOINT BUILDING

Award marks out of ten for your efforts.

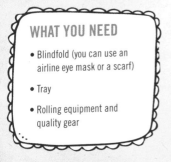

WHAT YOU NEED

- Blindfold (you can use an airline eye mask or a scarf)
- Tray
- Rolling equipment and quality gear

HOW TO PLAY

1 Lay out everything you need to build a spliff on a tray.

2 Everyone rolls a dice. The highest roller goes first.

3   Put the blindfold on the first victim and place the tray in front of them.

4   Help, laugh, or watch in dismay as they attempt to put together a decent blunt.

5   Award marks out of ten for appearance and smokability.

UP THE STAKES

This one is for serious tokers. Like the standoff at the OK Corral, you're in this for the long-term and you'll need butt cheeks of steel to stay in the game.

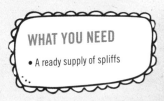

WHAT YOU NEED

• A ready supply of spliffs

HOW TO PLAY

1   Light up the first spliff, take a toke and pass it on to the next person. They have to take two tokes.

2   Keep passing it round, upping the number of inhales with each person.

3   When a player can't handle any more, they raise their hand and move out of the circle.

MARIJUANA MOVIE GAME

WHAT YOU NEED

• A collection of (preferably old) movies, made when smoking was positively encouraged on the big screen

• A ready supply of fat ones

HOW TO PLAY

1 Set up the movie and skin up some blunts.

2 Each time a character in the movie takes a puff on a cigarette, you pass round a spliff and do the same.

3 This also works for characters saying certain words, eating food, or slamming a door.

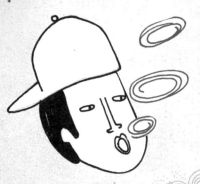

QUICK-DRAW DOOBIE

WHAT YOU NEED

- A timer—the one on your phone will do nicely
- Skinning-up equipment and a pile of cannabis

HOW TO PLAY

1 Fingers on the buzzers— it's literally who can build a blunt in the fastest time. But that doesn't mean rolling up a baggy, non-smokable excuse for a spliff. It has to be neat, tight, and smoke well.

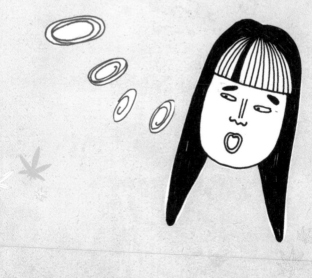

THE DOODLE GAME

Don't worry if you're no Picasso when it comes to drawing—the stakes are pretty level once everyone has been on the blow for a few hours.

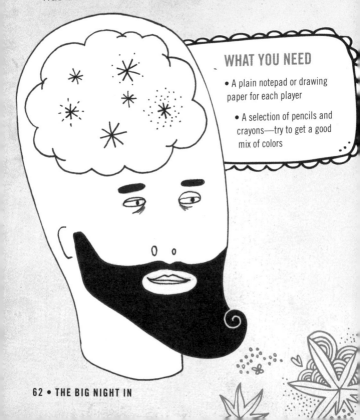

WHAT YOU NEED

- A plain notepad or drawing paper for each player

- A selection of pencils and crayons—try to get a good mix of colors

HOW TO PLAY

1 Choose someone to be "doodle master". They have to come up with a list of things to draw (try to keep it fairly simple, as you're dealing with stoners here).

2 Write each item on a small piece of paper and fold it in half.

3 Give one piece of paper to each player—they should look at it, memorize it (if they have enough functioning brain cells at that point), and then tuck the paper away so other players can't see.

4 The players then try to draw the item/person/animal on the paper. They should have a time limit of 30 seconds or 1 minute.

5 The first player should turn to the person on their right— if they guess correctly what they've drawn, both players take a hit of the spliff or bong. If the guess is wrong, both players miss out on the spliff and the game moves on.

THE "BIG NIGHT IN" CHECKLIST

You've blocked out Saturday night for pot pleasure-seeking. You've lined up some like-minded buddies, lined up some bud, and plumped up the sofa cushions in anticipation of a whole lot of sitting around. But before you get comfy, you'll need to get in some supplies—think of it like a mini world's end hunter-gatherer expedition. After all, you might not be capable of venturing outside for the foreseeable future, so you need to stock up on some essentials to see you through the high times and comedowns.

• **ROLLING PAPERS** Add a couple extra to whatever you think you'll need, in case it turns into a marathon session.

• **BEER AND SODA** One for the session, the other for the aftermath…just make sure you get plenty of both.

• **SALTY SNACKS** Chips, nuts, crackers, whatever floats your boat. Again, you can't have too many, so don't hold back at the grocery store.

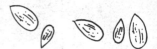

• **SWEET TREATS** You'll veer between salty and sweet cravings, so it's best to play it safe by stocking up on both.

• **MOVIES** Whether it's downloads or old-school DVDs, make sure you've got a good selection of viewing material.

Hours can quickly become days when you're on a bender and you'll need some background distraction to keep you going through the night. Check out our marijuana movie list on pages 66–67 for inspiration.

• **GAMES CONSOLES** Make sure everything's set up and ready to go; you don't want to be booting up systems, looking for controls, or charging devices when the effects of the holy herb kick in.

POT CULTURE

TOP TEN MARIJUANA MOVIES

1 *Fear and Loathing in Las Vegas* (1998)
The ultimate high times road movie, based on the classic
Hunter S Thompson novel.

2 *Harold and Kumar Go To White Castle* (2004)
Another road trip, but this one's a little more lighthearted.

3 *Dazed and Confused* (1993)
You'll wish you'd been at high school in the seventies when you
watch this with a reefer on the go.

4 *Jay and Silent Bob Strike Back* (2001)
Comedy cannabis capers abound in this movie about some stoners.

5 *Up In Smoke* (1978)
Every self-respecting stoner needs to watch this movie at least
once—it became an instant classic on release and is still top of
the cheeba film buff charts.

6 *Withnail and I* (1987)

The classic British stoner movie about out-of-work actors with a serious weed habit who leave London for a caper in the countryside.

7 *Homegrown* (1998)

Dope plantation workers have to find buyers for their crop when their boss meets an untimely end.

8 *Dude Where's My Car?* (2000)

The clue's in the title—a couple of stoners have a big night and forget where they parked.

9 *Saving Grace* (2000)

A cash-strapped widow turns her land over to cannabis plants to make ends meet.

10 *Easy Rider* (1969)

Straight from the era of hippies and hash cakes—the ultimate road movie that sees bikers travel the states.

TOP OF THE CROPS:
20 CHART-TOPPERS THAT MENTION MARIJUANA

1 "LEGALIZE IT" **(PETER TOSH)**

2 "MARY JANE" **(RICK JAMES)**

3 "BECAUSE I GOT HIGH" **(AFROMAN)**

4 "SWEET LEAF" **(BLACK SABBATH)**

5 "ONE TOKE OVER THE LINE" **(BREWER & SHIPLEY)**

6 "THE REEFER SONG" **(FATS WALLER)**

7 "DON'T STEP ON THE GRASS, SAM" **(STEPPENWOLF)**

8 "PASS THE DUTCHIE" **(MUSICAL YOUTH)**

9 "I LIKE MARIJUANA" **(DAVID PEEL)**

10 "CRUMBLIN' ERB" **(OUTKAST)**

11 "STONED IS THE WAY TO WALK" **(CYPRESS HILL)**

12 "CHEEBA CHEEBA" **(TONE LOC)**

13 "LET'S GO GET STONED" **(RAY CHARLES)**

14 "WE BE BURNIN'" **(SEAN PAUL)**

15 "HOMEGROWN" **(NEIL YOUNG)**

16 "HOW TO ROLL A BLUNT" **(REDMAN)**

17 "BIG SPLIFF" **(MURPHY'S LAW)**

18 "TAKE A TOKE" **(C+C MUSIC FACTORY)**

19 "GET HIGH TONIGHT" **(BUSTA RHYMES)**

20 "MARIJUANA" **(KID CUDI)**

TOKING QUOTES

"I have always loved marijuana. It has been a source of joy and comfort to me for many years. And I still think of it as a basic staple of life, along with beer and ice, and grapefruits— and millions of Americans agree with me."
Hunter S Thompson

"Herb is the healing of a nation, alcohol is the destruction."
Bob Marley

"Why is marijuana against the law? It grows naturally upon our planet. Doesn't the idea of making nature against the law seem to you a bit…unnatural?"
Bill Hicks

"I think people need to be educated to the fact that marijuana is not a drug. Marijuana is an herb and a flower. God put it here."
Willie Nelson

"I'd like to see the government back a program of research into the medical properties of cannabis and I do not object to its responsible use as a recreational relaxant."

Richard Branson

"Homer, I am getting really worried you are going overboard with this. We are out of clothespins, there are half-eaten cupcakes all around the house, and the curtains smell like doob."

Marge Simpson

"I don't consider weed to be any worse than having a beer."

James Franco

"I think pot should be legal. I don't smoke it, but I like the smell of it."

Andy Warhol

FESTIVALS

Marijuana is the perfect drug for festivals—pick a high-octane variety for head-banging near the stage, or a chilled-out bud for deep and meaningful fireside discussions with your buddies. There are literally hundreds of marijuana-friendly festivals around the world, but we've saved you the hassle of researching them all by picking out our guide to the top ten.

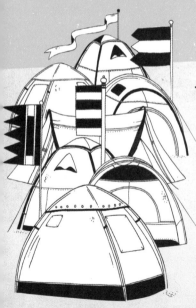

THE GREAT MIDWEST MARIJUANA HARVEST FESTIVAL (Wisconsin)

At more than 40 years old, this is the longest-running cannabis event in the US. Complete with music, lectures, and equipment vendors, this festival aims to promote the safe social use of the herb.

CANNABIS LIBERATION DAY (Amsterdam)

As the spiritual home of marijuana in Europe, it seems appropriate that Amsterdam gets to host a knees-up for the herb. This annual festival is a mix of music and talks dedicated to the international tolerance of weed.

THE HIGH TIMES CANNABIS CUP (Various)

The Cannabis Cup is the world's biggest cannabis trade show with events in different states that have legalized marijuana. With celebrity endorsements, music, and the unveiling of new varieties, this is a must-attend for serious stoners.

SOUTH PARK MUSIC FESTIVAL (Colorado)

Music and marijuana take the stage for three days at this festival, as herb lovers from around the world gather to show their appreciation.

NIMBIN MARDI GRASS (Australia)

If you find yourself Down Under in May, book a bus to Nimbin in New South Wales and join the joint party. What started off as a public demo against harsh anti-drug laws has evolved into a giant pot party, which pretty much sums up the feel-good factor of the mighty herb.

SPANNABIS (Spain)

Spain's huge cannabis trade fair is the most important event of its kind in the country and as well as some serious speakers, there's a whole load of music, paraphernalia, and weed-related exhibits.

420 FESTIVAL (London)

Although it's still illegal to smoke marijuana in England, for one day a year activists openly skin up and light up in London's Hyde Park. The idea is that with thousands more stoners than police, they can't all be arrested.

GYPSY JANE CANNABIS MUSIC FESTIVAL (Denver)

As the name suggests, weed is "high" on the agenda at this two-day hip-hop and high-times festival.

KUSH EXPO (California)

This may have the serious accolade of being the world's biggest medical marijuana event, but with glitzy awards, high-profile speakers, bars, and food, it's a festival by any other name.

BLAZE 'N' GLORY (California)

Expect plenty of wasted surf dudes at this new festival on the block that showcases the delights of the doobie to the accompaniment of an eclectic musical backdrop.

TOP FIVE GURNS

Gurning is the uncontrollable contortion of your facial features, and it's a sure-fire giveaway that you've overdone the cheeba and need to take some time out from toking. Over time, smokers tend to slip into a distinctive gurning style that helps their friends quickly spot when they've overdone it. Here's our top five gurns.

1 THE PROTRUDING LOWER JAW

This can either be a complete grimacing tooth display or a lopsided jaw shuffle that shows off a few of your pearly whites. If the music's on low, everyone will be able to hear your teeth grinding.

2 THE TEETH CLENCHER

Your teeth are on a mission to press together as tightly as possible and show no mercy to anything that gets in their way. If you keep up this gurn for too long, you'll have serious jaw ache the next day.

3 THE NEVERENDING CHEWING GUM

Start chewing on a strip of gum at your peril when you've been on the blow. When you're on a high, a few hours of chomping repetitively on gum will seem like just a couple of minutes. That means another comedown where you feel like you've been punched in the jaw.

4 THE SERIOUS EYEBALL ROLL

Your eyeballs take on a life of their own, as they wander off in different directions or disappear altogether so just the whites of your eyes are showing. This is often accompanied by head lolling, dribbling, and indecipherable speech.

5 DROOPY EYE

The eyes have given up altogether in this, the next stage on from the serious eyeball roll. The lids might flutter for a while as you try to fight the gurn, but soon they drop to a creepy half-shut state. Your only hope now is that you can make it to bed and sleep off your stoner state.

THE LITERARY LEAF

Casual links are often made between cannabis and creativity, but our list of literary caners shows that there might be some truth to the claim. Or maybe writers just have too much time on their hands...

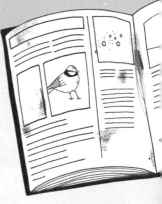

HERODOTUS

Though not exactly a household name these days, the Greek history bod was the first western writer to put pen to paper (or parchment) about pot.

ALEXANDRE DUMAS

The feted author of classic novels such as *The Three Musketeers* almost certainly got high when he penned about the high jinx of his heroes. As a member of the infamous Club des Hashischins in Paris (basically a weed appreciation society), Dumas was well placed to score the best quality gear.

BAUDELAIRE

It seems that French authors of a certain era shared a love of cannabis, and the poet Charles Baudelaire was partial to a pipe or two. However, he also liked the odd drink, and this was to be his eventual downfall.

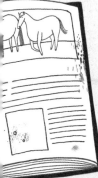

SHAKESPEARE

We know traces of cannabis were found in the great bard's backyard (see page 16) so who's to say he didn't inhale a little smoke to get his creative juices flowing. If so, then generations of school kids have been soaking up a lot of cannabis-laden literature.

HUNTER S THOMPSON

A prolific writer and drug connoisseur, Thompson liked to mix business with pleasure, as he referenced drugs with abandon throughout his works and enjoyed their recreational use as well.

MARIJUANA MUNCHIES

COOKING WITH CANNABIS

Smoking cannabis gives you an instant hit, but if you're looking for a buzz that creeps up on you like a panther then moves in for the kill, eating it is the way forward. To do this, you'll need to make a batch of cannabutter, which you can keep in the refrigerator or freezer until you get a craving for a culinary high.

Head to page 80 for the basic Cannabutter recipe, which will open up a whole world of caning cookery. Then check out The Badass Brownie on page 82 for the magic combo of chocolate and cannabis. If you've still got sugar cravings try the Vanilla Cupcakes (page 84) or super easy Gingerbread (page 86). Pot Popcorn (page 88) is the perfect accompaniment for a blitzed-out movie night, while Chili Con Cannabis (page 90) and Pothead Pizza (page 92) will fill you up and knock you out at the same time. Finally, head to the land of nod with a Caners' Hot Chocolate (page 94).

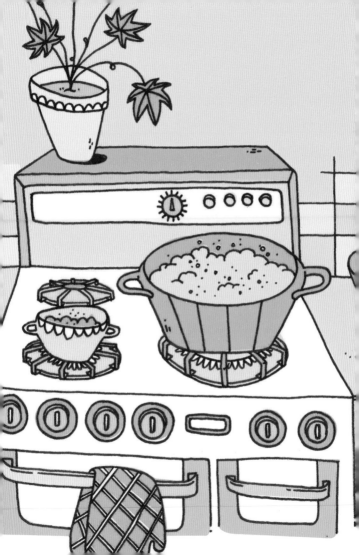

CANNABUTTER

MAKES 1¾ CUPS

1 oz top-grade cannabis
2 cups water
2 cups unsalted butter

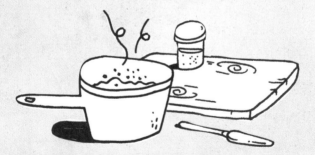

1 Grind the cannabis down to a fine powder using a strong coffee or spice grinder.

2 Pour the water into a heavy-based saucepan and bring to a steady boil over a medium–high heat. Once boiling, whisk in the cannabis powder until well combined, making sure there are no clumps and nothing is stuck to the bottom of the pan. Cover and simmer, stirring occasionally, for 1 hour.

3 Add the butter to the pan, cover again, and simmer gently for 1 hour more. Remove from the heat and allow to cool a little. If you want a bit more bite to your butter, repeat the simmering and cooling process twice more, but don't let it cool completely the last time.

4 Place a large square of cheesecloth over a bowl and carefully pour the butter mixture through the cheesecloth to strain the mixture into the bowl. Squeeze the cloth to extract as much of the butter solution as you can (this is what you want to keep, not the gooey leftovers in the cloth).

5 Place the bowl in the refrigerator and cool for at least 2 hours, or overnight, so that the butter separates from the water and sets at the top of the bowl.

6 Carefully cut or scoop the cannabutter out of the bowl and pat it dry with paper towels. Compress the butter into small, even-sized pieces and roll tightly in plastic wrap. Keep in the refrigerator or freezer until needed.

THE BADASS BROWNIE

MAKES 12–16 SQUARES

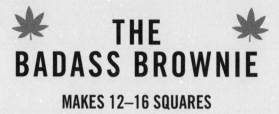

7 oz bittersweet chocolate, broken into chunks
14 tablespoons (1³/₄ sticks) cannabutter
(see pages 80–81)
3 eggs
1 teaspoon vanilla extract
1 tablespoon strong espresso (or 1 tablespoon
coffee granules dissolved in 1 tablespoon hot water)
1 cup superfine sugar
³/₄ cup all-purpose flour
¹/₄ teaspoon salt
²/₃ cup walnuts, roughly chopped
²/₃ cup pecan nuts, roughly chopped

1 Preheat the oven to 350°F. Grease a 13 x 9 x 2-inch baking pan and line the base with parchment paper.

2 Melt the chocolate and cannabutter together in a small bowl set over a saucepan of simmering water. Let cool for 5 minutes.

3 Beat the eggs in a bowl with the vanilla extract, espresso, and sugar until well combined, then beat in the melted chocolate mix. Add the flour and salt, and beat until smooth. Crumble the hash into the mixture—it can be in chunky bits if you want. Stir in with the roughly chopped nuts. Pour the brownie mixture into the prepared baking pan.

4 Bake the brownies in the preheated oven for 25–30 minutes. Be careful not to overcook them; the sides should be firm but the center still slightly soft. Let cool for 10 minutes before cutting into squares. Lift the brownies out carefully with a palette knife. Serve slightly warm with heavy cream, or cool completely and store in an airtight container between layers of parchment or waxed paper.

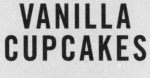

VANILLA CUPCAKES

MAKES 12

FOR THE CUPCAKES
⅔ cup lightly salted butter, softened
⅔ cup cannabutter (see pages 80–81), softened
¾ cup superfine sugar
Scant 1½ cups self-rising flour
3 eggs
1 teaspoon vanilla extract

FOR THE BUTTERCREAM
1⅓ cups unsalted butter, softened
1¾ cups confectioners' sugar, sifted
1 teaspoon vanilla extract
2 teaspoons hot water

1 Preheat the oven to 350°F. Line a 12-section standard-size muffin pan with paper cupcake cases.

2 Put all the cake ingredients in a large bowl, then beat with a hand-held electric beater until light and creamy. Divide the cake batter equally between the cupcake cases.

3 Bake in the preheated oven for 20 minutes or until risen and just firm to the touch. Transfer the cupcakes to a cooling rack to cool.

4 To make the buttercream, put the butter and confectioners' sugar in a bowl, and beat well until creamy. Add the vanilla extract and hot water, and beat again until smooth.

5 Spread the buttercream over the cooled cupcakes. Alternatively, put the mixture in a pastry bag fitted with a star tip and pipe swirls of buttercream on the tops.

GINGERBREAD

MAKES 24 SLICES

4 cups self-rising flour
1 tablespoon ground ginger
½ teaspoon baking soda
½ teaspoon salt
Generous ¾ cup light brown sugar
¾ cup cannabutter (see pages 80–81)
Scant ¾ cup molasses
Scant ¾ cup light corn syrup
1¼ cups milk
1 egg, lightly beaten

1   Preheat the oven to 325°F. Grease a 12 x 7½-inch baking pan and line the base with parchment paper.

2   Sift the flour, ground ginger, baking soda, and salt into a bowl. Put the sugar, cannabutter, molasses, and corn syrup into a saucepan, and heat gently until the butter has melted and the sugar has dissolved.

3   Pour the liquid into the dry ingredients together with the milk and egg, then beat with a wooden spoon until smooth. Pour the mixture into the prepared pan.

4   Bake in the preheated oven for 1¼ hours or until a skewer inserted into the center comes out clean. Let cool in the pan for 10 minutes, then turn out onto a cooling rack to cool. Wrap the cooled cake in aluminum foil to store.

POT POPCORN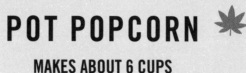

MAKES ABOUT 6 CUPS

1 tablespoon vegetable oil
⅓ cup popcorn kernels
5 tablespoons light corn syrup
2 tablespoons cannabutter (see pages 80–81)
⅓ cup roasted cashews, roughly chopped

1 Heat the oil in a large, heavy-based saucepan with a tight-fitting lid over a medium heat for about 1 minute. Add the popcorn kernels, cover with the lid, and shake gently to coat the kernels in oil. Cook until the popping sound stops, shaking occasionally.

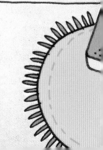

2 Pour the popcorn into a large bowl and set aside while you make the corn syrup coating.

3 Heat the corn syrup in a small saucepan with the cannabuter until melted, then stir in the chopped cashews. Cool slightly, then pour over the popcorn and toss until the popcorn is evenly coated. Put the popcorn in a serving bowl and tuck in.

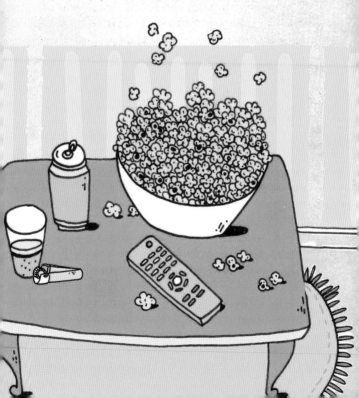

CHILI CON CANNABIS

SERVES 2

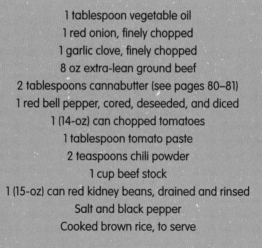

1 tablespoon vegetable oil
1 red onion, finely chopped
1 garlic clove, finely chopped
8 oz extra-lean ground beef
2 tablespoons cannabutter (see pages 80–81)
1 red bell pepper, cored, deseeded, and diced
1 (14-oz) can chopped tomatoes
1 tablespoon tomato paste
2 teaspoons chili powder
1 cup beef stock
1 (15-oz) can red kidney beans, drained and rinsed
Salt and black pepper
Cooked brown rice, to serve

1   Heat the oil in a heavy-based, nonstick saucepan over a medium heat. Add the onion and garlic, and cook for 5 minutes or until beginning to soften. Add the ground beef and cook for 5–6 minutes or until browned all over.

2   Stir in the cannabutter, bell pepper, chopped tomatoes, tomato paste, chili powder, and stock. Bring to a boil, then reduce the heat and simmer gently for 30 minutes.

3   Add the kidney beans and cook for a further 5 minutes. Season to taste with salt and pepper and serve with the brown rice.

POTHEAD PIZZA

SERVES 4

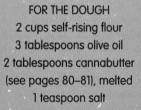

FOR THE DOUGH
2 cups self-rising flour
3 tablespoons olive oil
2 tablespoons cannabutter
(see pages 80–81), melted
1 teaspoon salt

FOR THE TOPPING
Scant ½ cup full-fat cream cheese
Scant ½ cup crème fraîche
2 tablespoons chopped rosemary
3 tablespoons olive oil
1 large onion, finely sliced
12 oz baby spinach
Salt and black pepper

1 Preheat the oven to 450°F. Grease a large baking sheet.

2 For the pizza base, put the flour in a bowl with the oil,
   cannabutter, and salt. Add a scant ½ cup water and mix
to a soft dough, adding a little more water if the dough is too dry.

3 Roll out the dough on a lightly floured work surface, into a
   round about 11 inches in diameter. Place on the prepared
baking sheet and bake in the preheated oven for 3–4 minutes,
until a crust has formed.

4 For the topping, in a mixing bowl beat together the cream
   cheese, crème fraîche, rosemary, and a little salt and
pepper. Heat the oil in a skillet and fry the onion for 3–4 minutes
until softened. Stir in the spinach and a little salt and pepper,
and cook for about 1 minute until the spinach has just wilted.

5 Pile the spinach onto the pizza base, spreading it out to
   about ½ inch from the edge. Place spoonfuls of the cheese
mixture on top of the spinach, then bake the pizza for
8 minutes or until turning golden.

CANERS' HOT CHOCOLATE

SERVES 2

2¼ cups full-fat milk
1 tablespoon cannabutter (see pages 80–81)
Scant ½ cup ground almonds
3½ tablespoons superfine sugar
2 teaspoons ground cinnamon
1 vanilla pod, split down the center
4 oz semisweet chocolate, broken into chunks

1 Place the milk, cannabutter, ground almonds, sugar, cinnamon, and vanilla pod in a medium saucepan and bring to a boil over a low heat. Take off the heat and let infuse for 20 minutes.

2 Pour the mixture through a very fine sieve into a clean saucepan, squeezing out the milk from the ground almonds.

3 Add the chocolate to the milk and stir over a low heat until the chocolate has melted. Serve immediately.

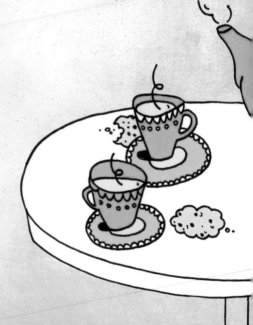

DISCLAIMER

The Publisher does not have any intention of providing specific advice and the content of this book should be used as a source of entertainment. All content contained in this book is provided for this purpose only and the reader's use of the content, for whatever purpose, is at their own risk. The views expressed in the book are general views only and the Publisher does not condone illegal activity of any kind.

The Publisher does not warrant or guarantee the accuracy or completeness of the advice or information in this book. In no event will the Publisher be liable for any loss or damage including, without limitation, indirect or consequential loss or damage, or any loss or damages whatsoever arising from use of the information in this book.